Hygge

Cozy Living The Danish Way (Denmark, Nordic Way, Contentment, Slow Down, Simply Living, Art of Hygge)

Astrid S. Nielsen

Hygge: Cozy Living The Danish Way (Denmark, Nordic Way, Contentment, Slow Down, Simply Living, Art of Hygge)

Table of Contents

1 - Introduction

What is Hygge?

Hygge trended in 2016. Books, articles, and social media buzzed about hygge. It was even shortlisted for Oxford Dictionaries' 2016 Word of the Year (post-truth eventually won as Word of the Year).

But what is hygge?

Tracing the Origins of Hygge

Hygge traces its roots from the Nordic culture, specifically from the happiest country in the world, Denmark. With the clamor for the antidote to restlessness, loneliness, and consumerism, people all over the world are seeking for concrete ways and role models on how to achieve happiness and meaning. This explains the hygge trend.

Pronounced as hoo-ga or hue-guh, hygge has no direct translation in other languages. The nearest words would be from Denmark's neighboring European countries: the Dutch word gezelligheid, German gemütlichkeit or gemütlich, Norwegian koselig, and Swedish mysig.

If ever, the closest English translation of hygge would be

cozy and convivial. And as Oxford Dictionary would expound, this sense of coziness and conviviality evokes and promotes a sense of comfort, well-being, community, and contentment.

Meanwhile, Collins Dictionary traced the roots of hygge from the 16th-century Norse word hugga, which means to console, and which is also the root word of hug.

Hearing from Danish themselves, the Denmark tourism webpage, Visit Denmark, succinctly describes hygge as a culture of cozy and intimate social gatherings that fosters a happy and relaxed feeling brought about by finding joy in the simple pleasures of life.

Hygge is about everyday togetherness that brings about that warm and fuzzy feeling inside. Hygge evokes a homey feeling of warmth, comfort, safety, and love.

Hygge also connotes a sense of intimacy stemming from a tight and snug atmosphere shared with loved ones, as well as a sense of safety from being sheltered and well-protected from harsh conditions outside specifically cold weather. This is understandable given the long and very cold winters in Denmark.

Again, Denmark tourism webpage perfectly describes this geographical roots of this concept. Hygge is the Danish coping mechanism for winter weather and challenges. During the winter months, Danish experience freezing temperatures, with 17 hours or 70% of their day in cold darkness.

Instead of mulling over and giving in to the so-called winter blues, Danes have grown to find their own spot of sunshine amid the cold, dark winter days. They choose to brighten up instead of feeling sullen or down.

In their minds, the cold and dark winter time is the perfect excuse to stay in, light some candles, curl up in soft couches, cuddle up with thick wool blankets, cup a hot chocolate in hand, or just watch the fireplace.

In the coldest winters and amid the strongest storms, they envelop themselves in warm atmospheres and connections to shield themselves against the harsh weather. Amid the miserable weather, the spirit is on fire with that warm and fuzzy feeling of love and comfort.

While the harsh-gentle dynamics of hygge is essential, it must be noted that hygge is actually not limited to winter, cold, or stormy days. Specific situations can be hygge too.

For instance, spending quality time with close friends can inspire a Dane to thank that friend for the hyggelig rendezvous, or meeting someone new and having an instant special connection would surely make a Dane say that it was hyggelig to meet the new friend.

Danes apply hygge in as many situations and moments as possible, as much as they inject hygge and its adjective form, hyggelig, in as many phrases and sentences as they can. Indeed, hygge permeates Danish culture.

2 - Exploring the Values and Focus Points Behind Hygge

Hygge is an art. It is a philosophy or way of thinking, a lifestyle or way of living, a feeling, an atmosphere, a particular situation, or a specific object that encapsulates the spirit of hygge.

In a scholarly dissertation, anthropologist Jeppe Trolle Linnet defined hygge as "a pleasant and highly valued everyday experience of safety, equality, personal wholeness and a spontaneous social flow."

Hygge is also about creating some sort of safe sanctuary while living a simple and authentic life, as described by Louisa Thomsen Brits in her book "The Book of Hygge: The Danish Art of Contentment, Comfort, and Connection". What this means is that the hygge sanctuary is not an escape from real life, but rather an extension and expression of it.

All these descriptions, definitions, and values of hygge center around authenticity, moderation, spontaneity, contentment, slowing down, and simple living.

These pillars or focus points make it different from the contract-like and hierarchical relations typical of work life, whether corporate or blue-collar. Hygge also differs starkly from formality and intensity.

Moreover, hygge contrasts with materialism, luxury, and consumer mentality bordering on hoarding. Hygge is healthy hedonism, as Signe Johansen coins in her cookbook and wellness guide "How to Hygge: The Nordic Secrets to a Happy Life".

In a way, hygge is finding joy in the ordinary, warmth amid the cold, and tearing down formalities to get to the heart of humanity.

In her article for Lonely Planet titled "Why I Love Denmark", writer Carolyn Bain wrote: "Hygge is social nirvana in Denmark: a sense of coziness, camaraderie, and contentment." It is about slowing down and living a simple life.

These pillars also shed light on the all-encompassing trait that hygge provides people who live the hygge lifestyle. Hygge is about how people maximize things like time, effort, and material possessions to express and experience love and warmth. In a way, hygge is similar with minimalism because it recognizes and prioritizes the essentials over the non-essentials.

It understands that life is not meant to be lived in the fast lane typical of a dog-eat-dog world, but rather it is meant to be enjoyed by slowing down and taking the time to light some candles and sip some wine with loved ones or perhaps just by having some simple tote-à-tête.

It understands that life is not meant to be complicated, toxic, or cluttered, but rather it is meant to be simple, flourishing, and pleasurable, filled only with things that make us happy, relationships that enrich us, and experiences that make us feel truly alive.

3 - Exploring Some Examples of Hyggelig Situations

To better understand hygge, let us example specific images, situations, and manifestations of hygge.

Imagine this: The first snow of winter just fell. You are strolling along the streets with your friends going home, laughing under the glow of the street lights. That's hyggelig.

Imagine this: Snow is falling heavily. You are sitting in the living room with your family, warming yourselves in front of the fireplace, sipping mulled wine, and talking about random things. That's hyggelig.

Imagine this: A storm is raging outside. You are snuggling with your spouse on the couch. Candlelight's dance in the soft wind coming from the tiny gap between the window and the windowsill. You sip hot chocolate and talk about how your day went. That's hyggelig.

Imagine this: A close friend invites you and your other friends over for a low-key dinner at her home. You enjoy a light and long conversation over a candlelit dinner of warm and hearty stew and a good bottle of red wine. That's hyggelig.

Peak hygge is described best by Meik Wiking, CEO of Happiness Research Institute, in his bestselling book "The Little Book of Hygge": It was Christmas Day. Meik and his friends were spending the holiday in a cabin in the snowy woods. They hiked in the snow.

When they returned to the cabin, they sat around the fireplace. They were wearing woolen socks and thick sweaters. One of Meik's friends thoughtfully wondered out loud if that particular moment could get any more hyggelig, to which another friend replied that it would be more hyggelig if it is storming outside.

Indeed, winters and storms are the most hyggelig seasons. Louisa calls hygge as "a cure for SAD or seasonal affective disorder".

Hygge is not a modern or recent thing. It is the very essence of Danish culture. In fact, if we look at the history of Denmark, it would be ripe with hyggelig elements.

Danish Film Institute has collated historical footage of hygge. Let us look at two examples.

First, let us look at a special occasion from a typical family.

It was Christmas of 1899. Peter Elfelt, Denmark's first film-maker, filmed his family while they were celebrating Christmas. They were gathered and dancing around the Christmas tree.

This hyggelig Christmas tree deserves its own description so let's focus on it. It is quite bare and basic. It is not the usual tree that is full of leaves and decorations. You can see the tree branches of this tree. It has candles and some simple hanging decorations. This tree is very hygge. It is not over the top. It just contains the essentials to make it a Christmas tree.

Now let us zoom in on the people. There are 6 adults, 1 kid held by the hand by the mother, and 1 baby carried by the father. When the family stopped dancing, they sat down, and one by one, they gave presents to the grandmother: a big box, a dog and then a plant. These gifts are very hygge too. They are living things. Hygge is about life and how life flourishes amid harsh conditions. They are gifts of hygge.

It was a very hyggelig moment for the Elfelt family.

Let us now look at an ordinary occasion from the royal family. One fine day way back 1955, the Royal Family sat down to have tea. Princess Benedikte entered the room leading Queen Ingrid by the hand. King Frederik and other 2 princesses followed. They took their seat in the plush couches.

The Queen prepared the drinks, and the eldest princess, Princess Margrethe, helped her. The other 2 princesses started helping themselves to the snacks of Danish pastries. The King spreads some butter on toasted bread.

When the Queen and Princess Margrethe finished preparing the beverages, they sat down to join the rest of the royal family. The King casually offers pastries to Queen. They too seem like a normal family enjoying a hyggelig moment. No servants buzzing about and tending to their needs.

All these examples of hygge, from past and present, have 2 common elements: first is cold weather, second is warm atmosphere shared with loved ones. This is the essence of hygge: how the warmth from genuine human interaction envelops you and keeps your soul afire, snug and safe from the cold and lonely weather.

In her New Yorker article "The Year of Hygge, The Danish Obsession With Getting Cozy", Anna Altman listed down other things that evoke hygge: fireplace, candles, lattes with latte art such as hearts, other warm beverages, wool, wood, slippers, rugs, blankets, socks, pastries, hearty soups, and other hearty dishes.

However, when we strip hygge down to these tangible elements, it can be too simplistic. While each of these items serves as a microcosm of hygge, each item in itself is not enough to create a truly hyggelig moment. As in other things in life, context is everything.

For example, while a tall cup of hot latte with milk-foam heart may remind a Dane traveling abroad of hyggelig moments way back home, it may not be enough to create a hyggelig moment right there and then, unless that person is drinking that hot latte in a hyggelig context, perhaps while chatting with a friend in the coffee shop.

4 - Other Danish Values Related to Hygge

Hygge also coincides with other Danish values. Let's explore three of them.

Privacy and autonomy

As Everyday Culture website points out, Danes value personal space and respect privacy. In this light, they do not snoop around and make presumptions.

Houses are very personal for them. Their residential spaces are extensions of their personal spaces and reflections of their personalities. Hence they do not invite themselves to another person's house. They wait to be invited. They do not make surprise appearances.

They also do not ask about a person's salary, house, and other material possessions. First, because they understand that this is none of their business. Second, because they do not care about these material acquisitions anyway.

Moreover, they avoid arguments as much as possible. Danes actually avoid showing extreme emotions, especially in public. They like social interactions to be smooth, casual, and relaxed. That said, they do not like being interrupted when they are talking. Interrupting them during conversations is akin to violating their personal vocal space or airtime.

Simply put, Danes mind their own business and consider it rude when other people, usually those from other cultures, bypass their sense of privacy. In the context of hygge, this means that a person shouldn't force himself/herself into a hyggelig moment with other persons. Hyggelig moments are not forced at all. It just springs freely.

Danes are able to hygge because they respect private spaces, spaces which are free from disturbance, stress, and negative vibes.

Understatement and modesty

Hygge encourages participation as opposed to the American habit of hogging the spotlight, as compared by Michael Booth in his article for The Guardian, "Hygge: Why The Craze For Danish Coziness Is Based On A Myth". This behavior also translates to Danish design as they favor functionalism and minimalism over flamboyance and flashiness.

We see this aspect in how hyggelig moments are structured. Snuggling in front of the fireplace at home instead of partying outside, eating dinner with family instead of eating outside in fancy restaurants, cooking meals at home instead of taking out quick oily meals in fast-food establishments.

Homogeneity and socially-rooted autonomy.

Global Utmaning positions Danish culture and hygge on the plane of being inclusively progressive vis-à-vis having socially-rooted autonomy.

Kay Xander Mellish, an English communications consultant in Copenhagen, described this particular idiosyncrasy of Danish culture in her podcast aptly titled "Why Job Titles Aren't That Important In Denmark." Kay observed that Danish "passion for equality" is evident in how Danish usually do not introduce themselves with their profession or work position, to the chagrin of other nationalities.

This sense of equality and unanimity is also embedded in their education system, wherein they put more value in group work instead of individual excellence.

This is very different from American culture of individualism. This is also different from Asian cultures such as Japanese and Chinese cultures that value community but still adhere to hierarchy. By contrast, Danes value community and equality. What sets it apart from communism is that Danes also value autonomy. That is autonomy in the context of community. This is Danish culture. It is also hyggelig.

5 - Criticisms of Hygge

Like other things, hygge has its pros and cons.

Middle-class mentality

It is often criticized as a culture of the middle class, bourgeois, or privileged segment. People argue that Danes can afford to hygge because they are safe and secure in their sociopolitical institutions. Or is it their hygge culture that enabled these safety nets?

Coercive or conforming

There are some foreigners who resided or worked in Denmark who observed that the homogeneous aspect of hygge tends to be coercive already. In other words, Danes expect outsiders to readily conform to hygge culture and they can also be quite intolerant of outside views. In this regard, Danes may come off as cliquish.

This pressure of social conformity is a disadvantage of hygge, especially for outsiders as well as for some Danes who prefer to embrace their individuality, uniqueness, or ambition, instead of going with the hygge flow. This brings us to the third criticism.

Intolerant of individuality and ambition

Hygge tends to shun and punish individuality. Since hygge values moderation and spontaneity, hygge may also seem to discourage and kill ambition, intensity, and passion. As some people commented, ambitious Danes would just leave Denmark and pursue their ambition elsewhere in the world.

Coming off as rude

In connection with cliquishness and conformity, Danes are also infamous for their shyness and disregard for formality. These facets may be construed as rude or tactless, but are simply by-products of their casual and private culture.

The Bottom-Line on Hygge

Danish culture of hygge is not perfect. No culture is. It has its perks and flaws.

Despite its quirks and idiosyncrasies, it has worked and continues to work for Danes. They have created a hyggelig community that gave rise to what Denmark is now: one of the safest, citizen-friendly, and happiest country in the world.

Who would blame people for looking up to hygge and to the Danish people as models on how to feel safe, flourishing, and happy?

6 - The Psychology of Hygge

Hygge fulfills basic human needs. But what needs?

Abraham Maslow discusses these needs in his psychological model, the Hierarchy of Needs. Maslow believes that humans are driven by various levels of needs, and he presents these needs in an inverted pyramid.

At the bottom of this inverted pyramid is the physiological or biological need. These are our basic human needs or what we need to survive. This includes food, water, shelter, warmth, clothing, rest, excretion, sex, among others.

The next level after this is the need for security or safety. This is also considered a basic need. We usually arrive at this secure state when we have a stable and reliable source of our biological needs, or when there is no or minimal threat of being deprived or robbed of these physiological basics.

While the first two levels are basic and physical, the next two levels are more psychological.

The third level is about love and belonging. Friendships and relationships fulfill this need for intimacy.

The fourth level is about self-esteem, and what fulfills this need is a sense of prestige and accomplishment.

The last two levels go beyond body and mind. They fulfill the needs of the heart or spirit.

Self-actualization is the fifth level. This is about achieving one's fullest potential. Some people call this manifestation and fulfillment.

The highest level is transcendence. This stage is about the need and desire to help other people maximize or realize their fullest potential.

How do we relate this with hygge?

Well, hygge takes care of the physical and psychological levels. It provides warmth and safety, intimacy and esteem. With these stages secured, the person can already attend to the higher levels of needs.

When the society and its institutions are arranged in such a way that they provide and support the basic needs of its citizens, the community turns out to be productive and happy, and the entire nation flourishes, amid environmental, geographical, and historical challenges and hardships.

Plants grow with sufficient light and water. Animals flock to sources of heat, food, and water. Humans thrive with warmth, care, love, and maybe a cup of a hot drink after a hearty meal shared with family and friends.

A culture of hygge fulfills these needs and makes people basking in its glow feel happy and content such that they are neither longing to be anywhere else nor wanting anything more than that hyggelig moment.

7 - The Geography of Hygge

While hygge can be achieved by anyone as it fulfills basic human needs, it is worth exploring in detail its country of origin. This will fill our curiosity about Denmark, but at the same time, there could also be lessons from the Danes that we can learn, or perhaps aspects that we can apply as we strive for hygge.

Manifestations of Hygge in Social Systems

Hygge is native to Denmark, a country known for its good social and economic policies and systems. Specifically, Denmark has:

- High standard of living

- Good social security system

- Universal health care

- Free university education

- Highest social mobility

- One of the highest per capita incomes

- One of the highest personal income tax rates

- High level of income equality

- Paid family leave

- At least 30 days of paid vacation leave per year

While it is good to its citizens, it also cares for businesses. This is a tricky thing to do for any state, and Denmark deftly does this by coming up with policies such as the so-called flexicurity, a portmanteau of flexibility and security. Flexicurity is described in detail by András Simonyi in his Huffington Post article "A Case for the Nordic Way".

With flexicurity, Danish employers can easily let go of employees during rough times, then hire new personnel as things return to normal. At the same time, flexicurity also provides reasonable benefit for the unemployed or those who have been let go by companies.

Moreover, flexicurity also has this system called "active labor market policy" that provides guidance, whether education or employment, to the unemployed sector. Denmark allots almost 2% of the country's GDP on this system.

This system is hyggelig. It provides a safety net, a safe sanctuary, for citizens and businesses alike. It gives them room to recover and to grow at their own pace.

Only a nation that values cohesion and consensus could create such a system. Flexicurity is a system-wide application of the essence of hygge. For András, while this model may not be universal or fit for other countries with different cultures, it can and should serve as an example of how to manifest positive cultural perks in governance and social systems.

8 - Manifestations of Hygge in Political Systems

Denmark also has a good political system. In 1849, the Danes abolished absolute monarchy and established a constitutional monarchy with a system of parliamentary democracy. The current political structure is able to yield effective programs for the citizenry as gleaned in its good socioeconomic programs previously mentioned. Moreover, Denmark is currently known for having the following:

- Protection of civil liberties,

- Democratic governance,

- Lowest perceived level of corruption in the world

- Efficient infrastructure.

9 - Manifestations of Hygge in the Environment

Denmark is also considered as one of the greenest and most energy efficient country in the world. This is not to say that Danes are environmental activities. On the contrary, they are quite nonchalant about environmentalism.

It just so happened that their hygge culture teaches about moderation, and this lifestyle of having just-right and consuming just enough shields them from the global trend of capitalism and consumerism, the by-product of which is wastage.

For Danes, environmentalism is about collective responsibility. It is also about staying true to the virtue of moderation and authenticity as innate buffers to environment-harming practices that we see in other wasteful countries.

10 - Manifestations of Hygge in Culture

Denmark consists of 400 islands, with only 72 islands populated. The country is bilingual. Danish is the national language, but they are English-proficient, as 9 in 10 speak English. In fact, more Danes speak English than German (only 6 in 10 speak German), even if Germany is just its neighbor.

With this, visitors to Denmark wouldn't find language as a barrier. However, staying in the country can be quite expensive for foreigners. For instance, 1 can (330mL) of Coke or Pepsi is 21 Danish Krones (DKK) or 3 USD in restaurants. With a high standard of living though, Danes are used to and can afford the prices of consumer goods.

Besides, with moderation as a virtue of hygge, you wouldn't find Danes gorging on soft drinks, junk foods, and other processed goods. With their Viking heritage and vast coastline, Danish diet is rich in seafood, although they also enjoy freshly-baked pastries.

Another aspect wherein hygge seems to be apparent is in how Danes shy away from religious and passionate topics. Indeed, they practice moderation not just in consumption but also in recreation and in religion. They prefer subtlety and simplicity over fanaticism and intensity.

As WikiTravel points out, Danes are generally agnostic people in the sense that they find it uncomfortable and even rude to inquire and talk about religion. Even religious symbols such as hijab, kippahs, and even religious statement shirts can make Danes feel awkward.

This cultural sensitivity must be minded by foreigners visiting or residing in Denmark, lest they alienate themselves. For instance, when someone sneezes, we normally say 'Bless you' but this is frowned upon in Denmark. Instead, say 'Prosit' or 'Gesundheit', preferably 'Prosit' because this is the Danish way, whereas 'Gesundheit' is German.

On a lighter note, Danes are proclaimed as the happiest people in the world. They also live in the most bike-friendly country worldwide. Aside from cycling, Danes are also into football, which is the national sport. They are also fans of music festivals and amusement parks.

In fact, Danes engage in outdoor and/or active activities such as biking, hiking, swimming, yoga, skiing, self-defense, boating, and running. They generally prefer outdoors to the gym. Moreover, they engage in these sports not just to improve their physical looks, but more so to be strong, empowered, and confident.

Their passion for outdoor activities is balanced with their equal passion for hyggelig moments at home.

Danes are quite the wholesome bunch, even when drunk. WikiTravel describes how Danes behave when under the influence of alcohol. Compared with other cultures wherein getting drunk is associated with violent behavior, Danes generally display overly friendly behavior when drunk.

This is because drinking serves a social purpose in Denmark of bringing people together in a hygge moment. Over-consumption of alcoholic drinks merely amplifies the natural predisposition of the people. Amid the culture of hygge, drunk Danes become cozier and more convivial.

This happy and active country also gifted the world, not just with hygge, but also with other famous products such as Lego game, Carlsberg beer, jewelry brand Pandora, dairy brand Arla, 1990s eurodance group Aqua, fairy tale writer Hans Christian Andersen, and sweet puff pastry product called Danish bread.

All these brands, products, and personalities display hygge

elements of minimalism (clean lines), functionalism (useful instead of ornamental), authenticity and quality, respect for tradition, right blend of playfulness and restraint, good blend of elegance and quirkiness, marriage of classic and modern, and combination of upbeat and mellow.

Bottom-Line on Hygge

From all these facets of Danish society and culture, we can see that Denmark's current systems, policies, infrastructures, traditions, products, and behaviors are hyggelig.

You see, it is not hygge per se that makes Danish people the happiest citizens, but rather how they have embraced hygge not just as a popular culture and passing thing, but as a philosophy that shapes their institutions and creations as well.

11 - Hygge and the Nordic Way

Studying and striving for hygge would also not be complete without a closer look at the bigger circle or the region wherein Denmark is situated in. Let's zoom out and examine the Nordic countries, specifically the Nordic Way. This will help us situate hygge for better appreciation.

Overview of the Nordic Way

Nordics cover 8 countries. On one hand, we have the five sovereign states. Three countries are from the Scandinavian Region, namely Denmark, Norway, and Sweden. The other two sovereign states are Finland and Iceland. The other three states comprising the Nordic countries are the associated territories, namely Greenland, the Faroe Islands, and the Åland Islands.

What do these Nordic countries have in common? They all have a culture that promotes good quality of living. We can call this The Nordic Way.

The Nordic Way is described best by Signe Johansen, author of the "How to Hygge", in his article for Evening Standard. Signe wrote that Nordic countries are "beacons of progress."

Signe cites that Nordic countries top the list when it comes to health (fitness level, low obesity rate, life expectancy), social systems (education, social security, health care system, public education system), gender equality, good environmental practices, and popular culture (food, architecture, design).

Perhaps we know of some people who just seem to win in life. They achieve so many things. They are a jack of all trades. They appear to do good things effortlessly. If these persons who win in life are countries, they would be the Nordic nations.

For Signe, these Nordic countries have undoubtedly hit the mark on the essence of daily living. At the end of the day, quality of life matters more than GDP and other economic indicators.

The History and Origins of the Nordic Way

This sense of culture developed throughout the years as a response to the environmental and economic challenges that Nordic countries faced.

The website She Does The City aptly describes this historical context of The Nordic Way and relates it to hygge. At some point in time, all the Nordic nations suffered from poverty. To adapt to limited resources and harsh environment and climate, Nordic ancestors developed a sense of thrift, pragmatism, endurance, and kinship or community support. These values are all embedded in hygge.

A similar value and concept with hygge is the Swedish concept of lagom, which loosely translates to moderation, which in turn is one of the aspects of hygge alongside authenticity and spontaneity.

She Does The City website further defines lagom as neither too little nor too much, but just about right. It is about choosing the reasonably moderate choices in life, with the understanding that too much or too little of anything can be destructive.

This sense of lagom is seen in other Nordic countries. In general, Nordic citizens neither skimp on food nor indulge too much. They have mastered the art of eating healthily and in moderation. Signe observed that Nordics love carbs because they believe that "life is too unpredictable to live in a state of puritanical abstinence."

While this is true, Nordics do not eat like there is no tomorrow. Their diet also consists of organic, home-made, or freshly-made food, and not the highly-processed and calorie-packed food from other countries such as in America. This is why obesity rate in Nordic countries are relatively lower compared to America.

Comparison of the Nordic Way versus Other Cultures

Other countries that closely mimics this sense of lagom includes Canada with its culture of moderation and Japan with their tradition of minimalism. Still, there are geographical and historical differences that make these countries unique from the Nordic way of lagom and hygge.

Another practice of the Nordic way and hygge is about being able to slow down amid the haste of life to appreciate the little things. One of the applications of this is fika, which is Swedish coffee break. For the Swedes, fika is not just about coffee, but also about cakes and chatting. Liz Connor, in her article for the Evening Standard, describes fika as "a moment to slow down and appreciate the good things in life."

Such philosophy involves acceptance and appreciation for

the present moment and current circumstances. And this contrasts starkly with other cultures that teach the value of dreaming and striving for more and more. For the sake of example, let's compare the Nordic Way versus the American Way.

First, the American Dream encourages and kindles individualism, while Nordics inculcate social rootedness. Second, Americans work hard to attain something better, but in the process, they arguably end up settling for something less ideal or perhaps something worse. On the other hand, Nordics appreciate what they have and make the most of these.

Such philosophy permeates these respective cultures, so much so that we can glean it even from their everyday diets. In an article for The New Yorker, Nathan Heller observes that the American diet is a microcosm or a reflection of the American life.

Let's look closely. The American diet is full of preservatives, flavorings, and substitutes for real foods. It is about burgers, fries, fried chicken, donuts, and other fried food, with a side salad. In the recent years, the growing trend of obesity has spurred health and wellness mentality, but in the form of energy bars and salad dressings.

By contrast, Nordic diet follows the balance and the practicality of the Nordic way. The Nordic fare is rich in seafood, meat, vegetables, and grains. Nordics like carbs and sweets, but they especially prefer the home-made or freshly-made version. They drink, but not to the point of violent intoxication.

Nathan concludes that perhaps for Americans with their Great American Dreams, Nordic life does not fall into their idea of how to live life, but in the end if Americans would just look closely, the Nordic life actually comes pretty close to the aspiration of the American dream—a happy and contented life.

For Nordics, their Nordic Way is good enough. At the end of the day, good enough makes them happy and abundant enough.

12 - The Art of Hygge

How can we achieve this philosophy and lifestyle of hygge? How do we achieve that delicate art of hygge?

In his book "The Little Book of Hygge", Meik Wiking, the CEO of the Happiness Research Institute, wrote about the Hygge Manifesto, which essentially lists down the 10 aspects of hygge.

The list has been picked up by influencers such as bloggers Laura Agar Wilson, Megan Cahn, Susan Baroncini-Moe, and Meena Hart Duerson. They have summarized Meik's list and adapted these to their own lives.

In this section, we will also summarize the main points of each of the 10 aspects to give you a better idea on how you can apply these in your own life.

The 10 aspects are shelter, atmosphere, comfort, presence, pleasure, gratitude, equality, harmony, truce, and togetherness. Let's go through each one by one.

Shelter

Shelter is a basic human need. It pertains not just to the physical structure, but also to the metaphorical shelter of having a tribe or a group of people who got your back.

For the Danes, it brings a sense of safety and peace of mind, that no matter what happens during the day, they can still go home at the end of the day, go home to a house where their loved ones are. It also brings a sense of security and comfort, that no matter how cold it is outside, their home is filled with warmth and love.

That shelter also serves as their private place where they can invite their friends over and entertain guests. In fact, they prefer to bond and hang out with their friends in their houses instead of eating out. They prefer chatting quietly among their compact social circle instead of partying out in big groups over loud music.

This communal sense of shelter is something that introverts and individualists may struggle to reconcile with. It is important to understand that hygge can be experienced even when alone, reading a book or engaging in a hobby.

Having said this, humans are also social beings, and even the most introverted and individualistic person in the world may find himself/herself clamoring for social connection every now and then.

At the end of the day, it is about having that delicate balance between personal space and emotional connection with other people. It varies from person to person, so find out what works for you.

Whichever level you choose though, may you find your physical shelter alongside your figurative shelter to provide you that warm and loved feeling, and that sense of safety knowing that you have a place that you can truly call home.

Atmosphere

This is in connection with the first aspect, shelter. Atmosphere is essentially the vibes of your shelter. Strive for cozy vibes in your physical shelter, and positive vibes with your social connections.

Susan Baroncini-Moe, in her blog post "Hygge: What It Is and How to Apply It to your Own Life to Create More Happiness", points out that atmosphere is perhaps the most superficial part of hygge. This is because the loose adaptation of hygge in the modern times calls for candles, sweaters, blankets, cushions, natural plants, dim lighting, among other elements.

While these elements are easy to achieve and serve as the

easiest way to enter hygge, there is a tendency to oversim-plify hygge by just boiling hygge down to atmosphere. Yes, atmosphere is an essential aspect of hygge, but it is not the alpha and the omega of hygge.

Atmosphere is okay, as long as we understand and realize that atmosphere is just a component of hygge and balance it out with other elements, as long as we don't expect to enter hygge with just a flicker of a candle, and finally, as long as we focus also on the intangibles and not just the tangibles.

With this caveat, what makes hygge atmosphere? Let's explore the common elements.

One, lighting. According to Meik, Danes like to create "soft pools of light" to mimic the "magic hour" or when the sun sets to pave the way from afternoon to evening. This time of the day, also known as dusk, is defined with its warm, soft, yellow-orange-red light with streaks of purple and blue. It's achieved by using dim lights and candles. As Meik points out, 28% of Danes light candles and tea lights on a daily basis.

Two, nature. Danes love nature and the outdoors. During spring and summer, they bask in the great outdoors, engaging in activities that make them interact with nature. Moreover, they like to bring nature indoors too. The presence of house plants, whether flowers, leafy plants, or herbs, can have a calming and relaxing effect.

It also adds authenticity and simplicity to space. It lends a feeling of home and safety, enabling dwellers and visitors to let their guards down. For Signe, nature also "allows you to reflect on the very essence of what living is about." It reminds you first and foremost that life can thrive anywhere, and that life is all around you. In the midst of this vibrance and liveliness, how can you not hygge?

Comfort

Hygge is about creating comfort. It is about seeking out what is comfortable for you and your tribe.

More than this, hygge becomes more hygge when you create comfort amid discomfort. As Meik said: "Hygge is possible only if it stands in opposition to something that is not hygge." Which is why there is that Danish notion that the harsher the outside condition is, the colder the weather, the stronger the storm, the more hygge you can achieve indoors.

Hygge is that contrast between warm inside and cozy outside, comfort within and discomfort out there. In this sense, hygge serves as a respite from daily strife. It provides relaxation amid the stress from daily life.

Hygge is not about attempting to change the world to fit what you perceive to be comfy. You can't stop the snow from falling or the rain from falling. Rather, hygge is about designing your surroundings to provide you comfortable shelter and atmosphere from the broader environment.

Comfort also comes from sufficient space or room to move. Danes veer away from clutters and decorative displays and instead favor things with meaning and stories. Louisa Brits talks about how Danes consider themselves as creator or producers, instead of mere consumers.

She wrote: "The things around us contain our stories and invite connection and conversation. Each home contains a symbolic ecology of objects and totems that speak of the lives of its inhabitants."

Aside from comfortable environment, it is also about that sense of comfort that allows you to be able to let your hair down and just chill, as the Americans would say. For Danes, this means wool tights, sweatpants, chunky sweaters, and knit or felt socks.

With these, we glean also that comfort is not something that Danes try so hard to achieve. On the contrary, comfort should be effortless. Otherwise, it would be contrary to one of the pillars of hygge, spontaneity.

Indeed, hygge and comfort should not be forced. As Louisa cautioned, hygge will elude us if we try so hard to capture and fabricate perfect moments.

So just chill, be comfortable, and let hygge follow.

Presence

Hygge is about being present, being in the moment, living in the moment. In a way, this is quite similar to the psychological and Buddhist notion of mindfulness, another concept, and lifestyle that is trending nowadays.

All hygge and mindfulness experts and enthusiasts agree that that easiest way to start these practices is by simply turning off your mobile devices, especially your smartphones.

The advent and proliferation of technology have made us

slaves to mobile devices. Even when we are with our family and friends, our hands automatically reach for our smartphones to check for notifications.

During lulls in conversation, we look at our phones to fill the silence that we fear would turn awkward, instead of letting the silence lead to comfortable companionship and eventually to another phase of the conversation.

It's as if we have this irrational fear of downtime that we want to fill the empty space of time with whatever we have on hand. Before we know it, we are scrolling through our social media feed or viewing memes and tuning out the conversation.

What about if we make the conscious choice of switching off our phones, putting them in silent mode, or just keeping them in our bags or purses? We do that when we watch movies in cinemas. Why can't we do that when we are with our family and friends?

Just immerse yourself in the moment, in what you are doing, in what your loved one is saying or not saying. Pay attention to non-verbals. Observe how they speak. Listen to what they have to say, without thinking of what to reply.

Listen to understand, instead of listening to react or reply. Just let the conversation flow.

Do not fill up lull moments and dead airs. Let the silence be a comfortable silence to just take in the hygge moment. Instead of turning inward, turn outward. Do not over-think, just be in that moment and enjoy.

As Louisa remarked, hygge involves respect and participation. When we stay in the moment, we show appreciation for that moment, and more importantly, for the people with whom we share that moment with. We make them feel that they matter so much that they deserve our full undivided attention and 100% engagement. We commit our time and attention to them.

In this sense, presence can also translate to thoughtfulness, so that you make your loving and caring presence felt even if you are not there. This could mean leaving a love note in the refrigerator, doing the dishes, watering the plants, doing the bed, or leaving a chocolate or a sweet treat for your office mate who has been sick or away. These little gestures show care, concern, and love.

These give us that warm and fuzzy hygge feeling, whether as

the giver or the recipient.

Presence also applies to solitary tasks such as reading a book, tending to a plant, or biking. You may be alone in these moments, but being present in the moment, or smelling the roses or taking in the view, instead of mentally wandering off to the past or future, can make a huge difference in how you experience that particular moment.

Pleasure

A lifestyle of hygge promotes enjoying the simple pleasures in life. Amid your day to day activities, take the time to pause and just savor the simple things in life.

Give yourself a treat, perhaps a hot drink, a sweet treat, or a creamy savory dish. It doesn't have to be extravagant. Danes would also stay away from artificial or highly processed treats, preferring natural and organic ones that are homemade or freshly-cooked. Indulge in your comfort food in moderation.

Pleasure also goes beyond food. Take pleasure in the company of people who make your spirit feel safe, alive, loved, and happy.

Gratitude

Thankfulness is also an essential aspect of hygge. Pleasure without gratitude is just worldly indulgence. Presence without appreciation is just compliance or conformity. And hyggelig shelter, atmosphere, and comfort are much more enjoyed and appreciated under the lens of a grateful heart.

Let's follow the hygge ways of Danes and just sit back, relax, and experience the moment with mindfulness and appreciation. Be grateful for the warm fire, the sweet Danish bread, the soothing drink, and the cozy and convivial feeling of being with your friends and kin. If you're alone, be grateful for the time to commune with yourself.

As Susan said: "It's when we're grateful for the simple things, the things that cost nothing, that we begin to notice and experience the true abundance of life."

This gratitude also stems from the feeling of being enough. That this moment right here is enough. You are enough. Meik wrote that hygge gratitude is rooted in the idea that: "This might be as good as it gets."

Some may say that this attitude sells oneself short. However, this is not settling down. Rather, it is appreciating life as it is. It is not about viewing life through rose-colored glasses or seeing the glass as half-full. Rather, it is experiencing the world via the soft glow of the candles, and seeing that the glass has water, and being grateful for things just being the way they are.

Be thankful for what you have now. Be thankful who you are with now. Be thankful for who you are now. You've got to be happy wherever you are. If you are not happy where you are now, you cannot be happy anywhere.

Equality

Hygge subscribes to "we over me" mentality which is very different with the American notion of individualism, with the capitalism concept of unique selling propositions and competitive advantage, with the Asian culture of top-bottom and hierarchies.

This is why Danes are not fans of job titles. They often introduce themselves only by their first names, which foreigners find puzzling, irritating, impolite, or too casual. They do not practice formalities and pleasantries because they look at people as equals. And when you view people in equal footing as you, you neither look up to them nor down at them. You just acknowledge their humanity alongside with yours.

This basic respect for humanity and equality manifests itself in how hygge practitioners make conscious effort to share activities, space, and time with other people. Hygge means sharing workload and tasks, as well as sharing airtime or storytelling time.

This means not hogging the limelight and not bragging about accomplishments, which presupposes that you spend time with people you don't need to impress or to patronize.

At the heart of this philosophy of evenness is the belief that everyone is equally worthy and valuable. It is acknowledging the light and warmth of love present in other people.

In a way, this is akin with the Buddhist and yogic phrase namaste, which translates to the light in me bows to the light in you, except that hygge namaste does not bow down or look up, it embraces and celebrates the light in other people, and letting the collective light warm each moment of connection. This is hygge.

Harmony

In line with equality is the other aspect of hygge: harmony. When there is no place for competition or bragging, when we believe that "we over me" is beneficial for the tribe, when we don't need to prove ourselves by putting down others or by bragging, harmony arises.

In music, harmony is the blend of tones and rhythm into something that we may call as music to our ears. For Danes, harmony is the blend of different people gathering together in cozy congruity.

People new to hygge make conscious effort to really listen to what each person has to say instead of listening to just respond. They ask questions to show that they are genuinely interested. They don't immediately counter or share their own stories, cutting off the limelight or airtime of the other person.

Harmony is like a chorus or a symphony. It is also like a group dance. In this sense, hygge is an art. Specifically, it is an art of blending and creating harmonious and genuine connections.

Truce

In relation with equality and harmony, hygge is also about truce. By truce, we mean no conflicts. Some chide hygge for this aspect because it is so ideal. The world is constantly changing, and with change comes conflict stemming from differences in beliefs and behaviors.

But what hygge teaches us is that, despite external conflict, we can find truce and peace within. Despite the world seemingly coming to different forms of war, we can find peace time if only we take time to venture into and embrace hygge.

Despite nature seemingly waging revenge versus environmental trespasses of mankind, we can come to terms with climate change when we make small efforts such as taking care of plants or not succumbing to consumeristic mindset resulting to wastage.

Truce also means no drama. When Danish friends and family come together, they rarely talk about politics or religion as these controversial topics can spur division and tension in the group. As Meik said: "Hygge is all about relaxed thoughtfulness. Save the talk about politics for another day."

This also differentiates hyggelig moments from hanging out sessions wherein people do extreme or daring activities such as who can drink the most shots of tequila. Hygge is more relaxed and non-competitive.

Hygge is also different from gatherings wherein people gossip a lot. During hygge moments, Danes do not engage in idle gossip. Rather, they focus on positive talks that uplift group spirit. They talk about ideas. Sometimes, they just stare thoughtfully at the fireplace, sipping mulled wine, taking in the cozy moment, and enjoying the companionable silence.

Togetherness

Danes do not talk about conflicts or drama. So what do they talk about? They talk about their day. They talk about happy times.

Indeed, hygge is about building relationships, and one of the ways to build relationship is by talking about shared narratives. Susan said: "Memories and storytelling become a way to share the ties that bind us. Nostalgia is a key component of hygge."

Hyggelig moments are filled with phrases such as 'Remember when we...' or 'Remember that time when...'

This sense of togetherness is not just apparent in verbal stories shared but in activities done by the group. Aside from sharing stories and memories, Danes also hygge by playing board games, watching movies at home, or just enjoying the fireplace and candles while the wind blows outside.

This sense of togetherness is also in stark contrast with the online type of togetherness that is common in this internet age. Nowadays, we can communicate with our friends via social media and messaging apps. These sites and apps make communication easy, convenient, and accessible.

While gadget-enabled communication is good when we are away or on-the-go, it is still good to have our share of in-person connections. When we connect offline, we get to experience the things that we would otherwise miss when talking via smartphones: voice, non-verbals, and cozy atmosphere shared with warm bodies instead of a warm phone.

Physical presence also prevents us from zoning out and allows us to enjoy the present moment more. When online, it is easier to just respond with an emoticon or smiley. It is also easier to misconstrue messages due to lack of tone and non-verbals. Friendships are easy to end and to fizzle out when we rely purely on online communication.

Hygge moments of togetherness preserve friendship. Togetherness fuel friendship. As Susan wrote: "Whatever you're doing, you're enjoying fellowship and coziness, in contrast to an increasingly angry world where friendships end at the click of the button."

This sense of cozy togetherness, alongside other Danish values, is what hygge is made of.

13 - Hygge, Contentment, and Simple Living

Contentment, moderation, and simple living are just three of the pillars of hygge, alongside gratitude and appreciation of the present moment. But what does it mean to be contented and to live simply?

Just Enough and Just About Right

From the lens of hygge, it is about being enough, experiencing enough, and having enough. It is about striking the delicate and much-coveted balance of just-about-right.

In her article for Lonely Planet titled "Why I Love Denmark", writer Carolyn Bain made the following observation about Danish notion of having enough that translates into an inclusive culture and thoughtful infrastructures and systems.

"While many countries are noticeable for the ever-increasing gap between the 'haves' and 'have-nots', Denmark seems to be populated by the 'have enoughs'.

"This egalitarian spirit allows the best of the arts, architecture, eating, and entertainment to be within easy reach of everyone. Indeed, the best catchword for Denmark might well be 'inclusive' – everyone is welcome and everyone is catered to, be they young, old, gay, straight, male, female, whether they travel with kids, pets or bikes in tow or with a mobility issue or handicap.

"Cities are compact and user-friendly, infrastructure is clean and modern and travel is a breeze."

To understand this from a technical perspective, let's look at the realm of research. In research, there are several types of rating scales.

On one hand, there is the Likert rating scale. This rating scale is the typical ones that we encounter when someone interviews us and asks, 'How satisfied or dissatisfied are you with so and so?' To which we have to choose from 5 options, usually from a rating of 1 which means 'Not satisfied at all' to a rating of 5 which means 'Very satisfied'.

On the other hand, there is what we call as sensorial ratings or just-about-right or JAR rating scales. This is usually asked during product testing. The question goes like, 'What do you think about the sweetness of this product?'

To which we have to choose from 3 options, from rating of 1

which means 'Too lacking in sweetness compared to what I want', to a rating of 2 which is the ideal one that means 'Just about right sweetness, no need to change level', and to a rating of 3 which means 'Too sweet compared to what I want'.

Concepts such as Americanism, consumerism, capitalism, and materialism are all akin to Likert rating scales. We always want to get the highest possible rating. We want to get to the top. We want to be the best. We want people to be delighted with our personal brand. We want to impress people by being over the top.

By contrast, hygge is about striking that sweet balance. Hygge belongs to the realm of just-about-right. This is also a good metaphor because hygge is also a sensorial thing. When we hygge, we listen to our senses and to our guts to arrive at hygge or balanced moments.

And once we achieve that just-enough state, we get to be attuned with what we really want, and in that level, we just feel happy and contented. We don't want to change a thing.

Minimalism and Prioritizing the Essentials

Another idea that trended over the recent years is minimalism as advocated by Marie Kondo, Joshua Becker, Joshua Fields Millburn, and Ryan Nicodemus, to name a few influencers.

The essence of minimalism is encapsulated in three words by Robert Browning in his 1855 poem entitled Andrea del Sarto: The Faultless Painter. Robert wrote: "Less is more."

While minimalism and hygge are distinct movements, they share the similar principle of acknowledging and focusing on the essentials instead of the non-essentials. Essentials being building and nurturing relationships, whereas non-essentials are material acquisitions and worldly desires such as popularity, reputation, distinction, accomplishment, and physical appearance, among others.

This is also connected with the notion of having enough. There are some people who think they just need to organize their lives. So they buy planners, organizers, filing cabinets, folders, storage bins, etc. They hold on to their materials possessions for the sake of nostalgia and display.

They think they need more than one set of television or nice antique bowls that they don't use anyway. In the end, these things just accumulate and end up as clutter. But what if they just let go? What if they just realize that they don't need to hold on to these material acquisitions?

"For the longest time, I thought I needed to be more organized. Now I know I just needed less stuff," Alysa Bajenaru, dietitian and blogger, shared on her blog.

Similar with minimalism, hygge is the antithesis of hoarding and perpetual accumulation. Some may think that hygge is markedly different from minimalism because they think hygge elements such as candles and woolen socks are excessive. But it is only excessive if you accumulate things that serve no purpose or have a redundant purpose.

It is also worth pointing out that minimalism does not equate bare and boring. Minimalism is not poverty. Rather, minimalism is all about mindful placement. In hygge, candles and woolen socks are not just for display but they serve the specific purpose of lending a cozy atmosphere to the place wherein one can spend quality time with loved ones.

As Nicholas Burroughs, graphic designer, said: "Minimalism is not a lack of something. It's simply the perfect amount of something." So is hygge.

This perfect amount of something as a quality of both hygge and minimalism is also described succinctly by media activist Duane Elgin: "The intention of voluntary simplicity is not to dogmatically live with less. It's a more demanding intention of living with balance. This is a middle way that moves between the extremes of poverty and indulgence."

Simple living is all about living with purpose and love. It is about being happy and thankful for what you have, with who you are, and with whom you are with. It is appreciating the present moment and being content. When you are contented, you let go of expectations, assumptions, earthly desires, emotional baggage, clutter, and competition.

With the warmth of connection and purpose, you relish the moment and thank the universe for that moment in time. This is minimalism. This is presence and gratitude. This is hygge.

14 - Hygge and Authenticity

We live in a world wherein narcissism and self-promotion are easy and sometimes even encouraged. We like to post selfies and food shots, as well as status updates. This is not to say that self-aggrandizement is a product of the internet age. This has existed even pre-digital era. People's penchant for bragging and gossiping just got louder in the context of digital culture.

Amid this, it is also easy to compare ourselves with people sharing about their seemingly perfect and grandiose lives online. It can breed discontent if we are not self-aware and grounded. It can lead us to think about what we lack instead of what we have.

You see your "friends" traveling around the globe, getting engaged, getting married, having babies, eating delicious food, cooking picture-worthy dishes, and experiencing the world like you are not experiencing. And it makes you think, 'shocks, my life is so boring' and you ignore your friends in real life and just mope around all day, thinking about what could have been and what will never be.

This is NOT hygge.

When you live a life of hygge, your focus is not on your online life, but on your real life, your life offline. You don't pose pictures and status updates on your social media to impress people. You just do your own thing and let your life speak for itself.

Humorist Robert Quillen further sheds light on what authenticity is not: "We buy things we don't need, with money we don't have, to impress people we don't like."

Hygge, with authenticity as its pillar, only seeks essential things that support connection with people it holds dear.

15 - How to Live a Simple Life of Hygge and Contentment

There are many tips on how to apply hygge to live a simple life, but one of the most practical ways is given by journalist and media expert Shannon L. Bowen, in her article for Signature Reads entitled "6 Steps to Achieving Hygge, the Danish Art of Contentment and Comfort".

First and foremost, Shannon reminds us that while material things can contribute to hyggelig moments, they are not the be-all and end-all of hygge. You do not need material things to feel hygge.

Remember that hygge is born out of community, resourcefulness, and appreciation. Material things such as a cup of tea, a wooden table, and a knitted sweater are just physical manifestations of hygge. More important are the intangibles.

Having said this, Shannon proposed six ways on how to apply hygge in our daily lives. Her list is practical applications as opposed to the value-based list from Hygge Manifesto. However, the methods she proposed still contain the pillars and values of hygge as described by other authors. Let's now explore these steps.

Think of others instead of being absorbed in yourself

When we think about ourselves too much, we fail to engage fully with people around. When we are too much absorbed in our inner world, we fail to appreciate and participate in the outside world.

Introversion and introspection are necessary components for a rich inner world and holistic growth. But too much of anything can be destructive and counterproductive.

Even the most introverted person needs some time to spend with people. It keeps us grounded. It comforts and consoles us. It keeps us contented instead of feeling stressed, anxious, and bottled up.

Focusing on other people is also a humbling endeavor. We realize that the world does not revolve around us and that people do not think about our weaknesses and shortcomings as much as we think they do.

We also start to appreciate them for who they are in their entirety, instead of judging them when they fail our expectations and assumptions. So let's get off our high tower of

overthinking and go out into the real world of human interactions.

Out in the real world is where we get the opportunity to treat others with sincerity, kindness, thoughtfulness, and generosity. We realize that we are not responsible for ourselves alone, but for other people too. We start to genu-incly care and reach out to other people. We got their backs, and in turn, they got our backs too.

As Louisa Brits wrote, when we are happy and contented deep inside, when we feel enough, we reach out to other people not to complete us but to genuinely love them. We feel responsible for them in a mutual manner, neither de-pendent nor dominating, neither clingy nor manipulating.

Indeed, hygge is about reciprocity and mutual caring.

Transform everyday activities into daily rituals, and relish them instead of running on autopilot

As we go through our everyday lives, we tend to go on auto-pilot. We just do things out of habit, mindlessly going through the day just like what we do every single day.

Hygge teaches us that we can find joy in routine and that occasional break from monotony. Shannon suggests enjoying a warm bath instead of a quick shower. Or perhaps liven up your dinner table by putting a vase with fresh flowers as a centerpiece.

Or dim the lights and put up some scented candles while you sip your decaffeinated coffee before going to bed. Or instead of just spritzing cologne and going your way, why not take time to inhale that dab of fragrance on your wrist for a couple of seconds?

As Louisa said, rituals transform the commonplace into heartfelt. Even the most mundane task can be enjoyed on a different level if we do it with mindfulness, presence, purpose, and love. Remember: we are humans, not robots.

Light some fire and kindle the flame

As mentioned throughout this book and in other books about hygge, warmth, both literally and metaphorically, is the primary essence of hygge.

As Shannon points out, the warm and lively glow of the fire brings people together, be it a bonfire or a candle, a fireplace or a streetlight.

So seek warmth, in whichever physical form. Be it fire or warm soup. Also, seek warmth from social connections. Kindle the flames from these sources of warmth and you're set for life.

As Louisa expounds, hygge is about creating a circle of life, gathering a close-knit group of people around a fire to celebrate the moment of warmth, security, and connection. There is a primal sense of comfort about gathering around a bonfire on a cold dark night with good friends.

Fourth, find and renew the connection with nature by caring for plants and animals, or just by spending more time with nature, whether indoor or outdoor.

Louisa also wrote that Danes are rooted deeply in nature and rural landscape. Hence, even in the modern Danish society wherein, people live in apartments and modern houses, they still make time to engage in outside activities. They also like to bring nature inside their houses by tending to indoor plants or houseplants, and leaving the windows open on days when the weather is nice.

Other cultures can adopt hygge by doing picnics in parks, taking nature walks, camping, and gardening. Louisa talks about how gardening reminds us of our place and role in the natural world, how touching soil allows nature to touch our soul, and in that connection, we reflect on our being and humanity. Hygge is not just mutual caring for our fellow humans, but mutual caring with other living creatures and with the natural world in general.

It makes us more caring and loving, in the same way that pets do. In the course of your daily life, just ensure that you get to spend quality time not just with people, but with nature too, whether plants or animals.

Examine and de-clutter your environment, then curate

This aspect is essentially minimalist. It requires us to de-clutter, which means to let go of things that do not serve a real and unique purpose in our lives. It means letting go of things so that we have more space for things that really matter.

It is not about leading a monkish life of non-possession, it just means having only just enough and being content with that. Minimalism proponent Joshua Becker remarked: "Minimalism is not that you should own nothing. But that nothing should own you." The same can be said for hygge.

As Louisa said, we must keep things only when they are useful, or when they contribute something to our well-being. When we do this, we live a simple and hygge life. Hygge is all about mindfulness, harmony, and balance. It is neither control nor mess, neither obsessive-compulsive nor disorderly.

So de-clutter, let go, and be mindful of the things you keep and the things that you buy. Keep and acquire only the things that contribute to hygge, only the things that speak to your soul and/or express your spirit.

Be present

Real-time is the in thing in this internet age. In this modern age, we want things fast, at the speed of light. We have fast-food, fast-printing, express lane, and other things that save us time. Why then do we feel that we still lack time? Why are we stressed, vexed, and rushed?

Why don't we slow down? Hygge provides an antidote to this fast-paced modern world. It is similar to meditation and mindfulness, but more sensorial than process-based. Again, Louisa put this beautifully when she said that hygge is more about noticing rather than contemplating. It is about being present and being aware of the moment.

Amid this world of uncertainty, real-time technology, and capitalism, there is merit in applying some hygge in our lives, whether it is adopting stray pets, planting herbs, inviting friends over for a candlelit dinner instead of dining out, or just doing a simple and kind gesture to a neighbor.

How about you? How do you hygge?

16 - Hygge, Slowing Down, and Cozy Living

Hygge trended last 2016, the year considered as the worst year due to various global happenings especially in politics. With so much chaos and uncertainty, people continue to search for happiness anchors.

The Danes have long held on to their hygge tradition as a cure for bad weather and bad times. The world is on to something as they discover the magic of hygge.

Slow down

Hygge does not only advocate for a simpler lifestyle, but also for slower lifestyle. It encourages people to slow down, not just to take the time to smell the flowers, but to tend to the flowers too.

Slowing down is best encapsulated in the reflection of entrepreneur Derek Sivers, as featured in Timothy Ferriss's book Tools of Titans.

Derek used to ride his bike in a sandy bike path that goes for 25 miles. He would bike really fast and hard, huffing all the way, and ending up red-faced at the end. It took him about 43 minutes every time.

However, as time went by, he noticed that he was starting to lose enthusiasm to bike because he was dreading the pain. He felt burned out.

So one day, he just decided to go slow. He biked on the same path, but instead of trying too hard, he just took it easy. He stood up in his bike instead of crouching down. He looked around instead of down.

He saw the ocean. He saw dolphins jumping up and down the ocean. He noticed a pelican. He felt a pelican pooped on him. He found it funny. He had a leisurely bike ride. It was utterly pleasant. He did not huff. His face was not red.

In the end, he looked at his watch. It took him just 45 minutes.

The experience was purely profound for Derek. All those huffs and puffs, his red face, his pain, and stress—all these were just to save 2 minutes. He decided that the 2 extra minutes are not worth it. He now knows when enough is enough.

He applies this principle to life. Now, he stops himself before he feels burned out. He pauses before he hits that point of being too stressed.

When was the last time you slowed down? When did you try to maximize your efforts to save 2 minutes, making you dread the effort and feel too stressed?

Why are you hesitant to slow down? Some people would say it is slacking off. But really, why are you rushing about any-way? What's the rush? Know your threshold. Know that there is still tomorrow. Know when to chill and relax.

Danish writer Hans Christian Andersen once quipped: "Enjoy life. There's plenty of time to be dead." Indeed, this is a very Danish and hyggelig thing to say. This is because Danes believe in not taking themselves too seriously. They just let things be. They just let the light shine amid the dark, cold night.

This reminds us of the 1970 song "Let It Be" by English rock band The Beatles, the lyrics of which goes:

"And when the night is cloudy

There is still a light that shines on me

Shine until tomorrow

Let it be"

It is comforting to know that hygge is actually more universal than we think. It is just a matter of living simply and letting things be. You can start by cozying up.

Get warm and cozy.

But how do you cozy up?

In her article for Telegraph UK entitled "Say Hello To Hygge: The Danish Secret To Happiness", Maria Lally summarized some points proposed by Helen Russell in her book "The Year of Living Danishly: Uncovering The Secrets of the World's Happiest Country".

Celebrate and find joy in the simple things

Savor each sip of your coffee and that rich cake. Find shape in the clouds. Walk slowly, taking in each sight, sound, and smell that you encounter. Listen, really listen, to people as they talk.

Reframe rainy and snowy days, literally and figuratively

Embrace whatever the weather is and don't let it dictate your mood. Maria suggested changing our mindset. Treat winter days as a season to gather and cuddle in front of the fire. Consider rainy days as a good excuse to stay in and read that new book with a cup of hot chocolate in hand.

Make chilly evenings as a reason for cooking hearty stews with your family. The old adage says that misery loves company, but the Danes would say, miserable times get better with company and hygge.

Consume real food and eat in moderation.

Nowadays, we get health enthusiasts buzzing about eating clean, yo-yo dieting, etc. Maria proposes that we forget this #eatclean and instead #eathygge.

Danes eat comfort food like what grandmothers and mothers cook. They like hearty meals, fatty and sweet food. What they are not fans of is highly-processed food that is typical of the American diet.

Danes do not control their eating. They don't overeat either. They just eat in moderation. They follow their guts. And the fact that obesity is low in Denmark is a sign that this is working for them.

So ditch your diets and just hygge your way to a healthier lifestyle.

Create and maintain a happy and cozy home.

Maria and Helen observed that houses in Denmark are havens of hygge. Common elements are leather, wood, sheepskin, cushions, and wool, among others.

And what is the effect of having these hyggelig elements? It reminds them of hygge and coziness. Surrounding yourself with beautiful things also makes you happier, as revealed by scientists from the University College of London. Beautiful things stimulate dopamine, the happiness hormone. It is no wonder then why simply walking into a Danish home is enough to instantly get that dose of hygge.

Beauty, as they say, is in the eyes of the beholder. So if Danish furniture is not really your thing, then don't force it. Just create an atmosphere that you and your loved ones consider happy, cozy, and comfortable. Personalize it. It's your space anyway. Do what makes you happy. That's the hygge spirit.

Prioritize your loved ones

Sure, you can be cozy by being alone. But no man is an island. You need love and warmth from human connection too. Know that hygge is not about candles and plush cushions. More importantly, hygge is about connection and love.

So come on, get cozy with your friends and family, and start to feel hygge shine its light in your life.

Thank You

As we reach the end of this book, I want to say thanks for reading this book.

I want to get this information out to as many people as possible. If you found this book helpful, I would greatly appreciate you leaving me a review. This helps others find the book as well.

Disclaimer

This document is geared towards providing exact and reliable information in regards to the topic and issue covered. The publication is sold on the idea that the publisher is not required to render an accounting, officially permitted, or otherwise, qualified services. If advice is necessary, legal, financial, medical or professional, a practiced individual in the profession should be ordered.

This information is not presented by a financial or medical practitioner and is for entertainment, educational and informational purposes only. The content is not intended as a substitute for professional medical advice, diagnosis, or treatment. Always seek the advice of your physician or other qualified health care provider with any questions you may have regarding a medical condition. Never disregard professional medical advice or delay in seeking it because of something you have read.

The information provided herein is stated to be truthful and consistent, in that any liability, in terms of inattention or otherwise, by any usage or abuse of any policies, processes, or directions contained within is the solitary and utter responsibility of the recipient reader. Under no circumstances will any legal responsibility or blame be held against the

www.ingramcontent.com/pod-product-compliance
Lightning Source LLC
LaVergne TN
LVHW010655200726
843507LV00011B/1883